Baby tips
for grandparents

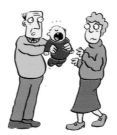

Simon Brett
Bestselling author of *How to be a Little Sod*

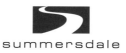

summersdale

BABY TIPS FOR GRANDPARENTS

Summersdale Publishers Ltd
46 West Street
Chichester
West Sussex
PO19 1RP
UK

www.summersdale.com

Printed and bound by Tien Wah Press, Singapore

ISBN: 1-84024-490-9
ISBN: 978-1-84024-490-8

Contents

Introduction

You may think being a grandparent's easy, that all you have to do is sit back and enjoy watching the development of another generation. But being a grandparent brings all kinds of new challenges. It puts new stresses on your relationship with your children and it's also a diplomatic minefield. You'll find, in your new role, you spend a lot of time biting your tongue to avoid saying the wrong thing. Oh yes, it's tough.

How fortunate then that you have this small book of advice to guide you through the choppy waters ahead.

Rocking the Cradle

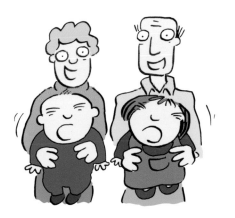

Before the baby's born

Try not to ask: 'Should you be doing that in your condition?'

A grandmother-to-be should try to avoid turning into a primitive Wise Woman, dangling keys or needles over the bump to predict gender.

When its parents
announce the name
they have chosen
for your grandchild,
try not to wince – or,
even worse, giggle.

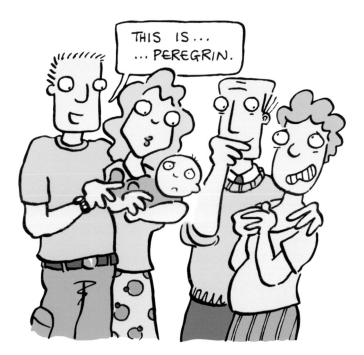

Don't suggest lending your books on pregnancy to the mum-to-be. Fashions in such matters have changed, and the gurus whose advice you followed have been long since discredited.

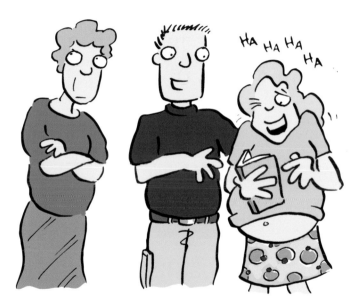

If you want to retain any friends, try occasionally to talk to them about something other than the impending birth.

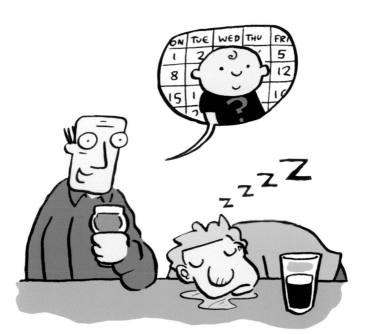

Don't say to first-time parents-to-be, 'You'd better make the most of your freedom now. You won't have any social life once the baby's arrived.' It's true, but there's no point in depressing them before it happens.

What not to say as a grandparent

Avoid sentences which begin 'I always gave you…' and end '… and you've turned out all right.'

Try to avoid saying,
'In our day we just
got on with it.'

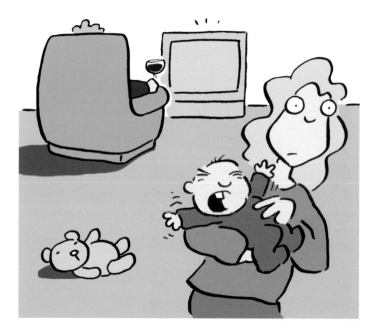

Or, 'The odd non-organic vegetable never hurt anyone.'

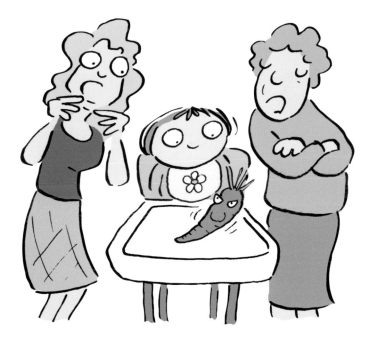

Or, 'We didn't bother with any of that nonsense when you were a baby.'

Never say to a first-time mum-to-be: 'You won't have time to be so fussy with the next one.' While undoubtedly true, it is not what she wants to hear.

When your grandchild
misbehaves, do
not overreact by
announcing, 'I'm going
to change my will.'

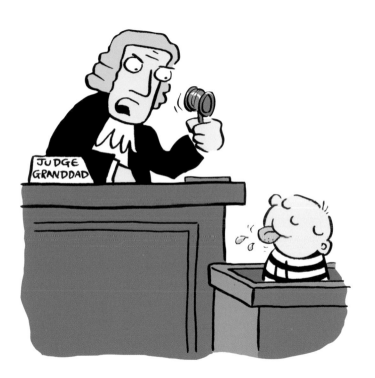

It is inadvisable to say to the parents of your grandchildren, 'You spoil that child.' But if they say it to you, just smile with infuriating smugness and say, 'Yes.'

Advice to grandparents
contemplating saying
how much better
children were brought
up in their day: Don't.

Unavoidable Clichés

'I'm so much more
relaxed with them than
I was with my own.'

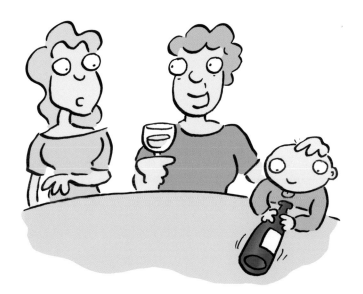

'The trouble is, these days
children aren't allowed
to have a childhood.'

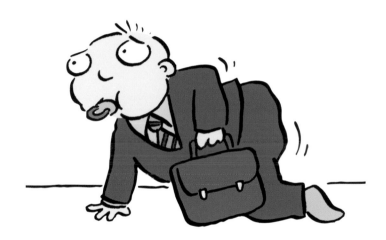

'It seems no time at
all since their parents
were that age.'

'Ooh, look, the baby's more interested in the wrapping paper than the present!'

'Well, you're
eating for two.'

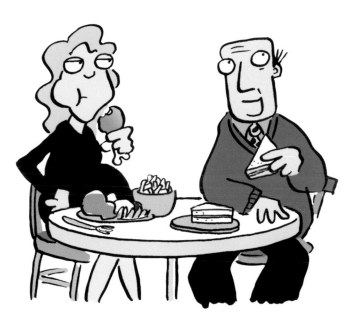

'The good thing is you can give them back at the end of the day.'

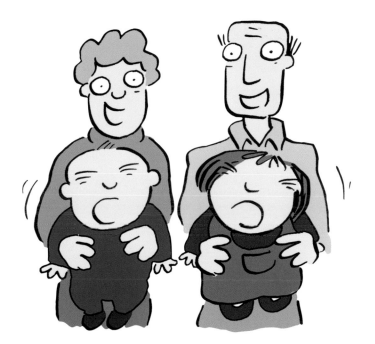

General Rules

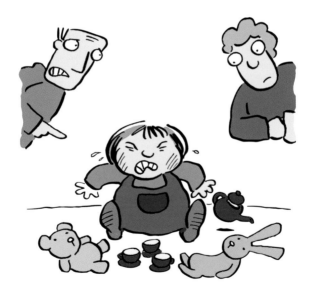

Top Tips

Never pretend you're too young to be a grandparent. The contradictory evidence is there in the cot.

Always deny that there is any rivalry between you and the other set of grandparents. Though, of course, there is.

Do not get down on the floor to play with your grandchild unless you are confident you will be able to get up again without assistance.

Even though you've failed
with two generations,
don't try to realise your
dreams through a third.

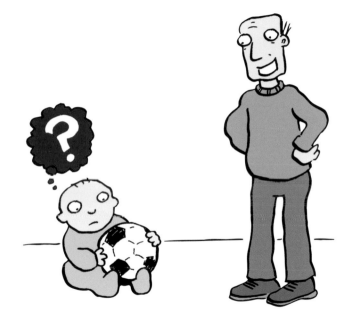

You will meet a lot of
pathetic souls labouring
under the delusion that
their grandchildren
are more beautiful and
intelligent than yours.
Ignore them – obviously
they are wrong.

When your grandchildren come to stay

When its parents leave your grandchild at your house, there are bound to be tears. But you just have to pull yourself together.

Grandchildren will never remember where to put their toys away but they'll always remember where you keep the crisps and biscuits.

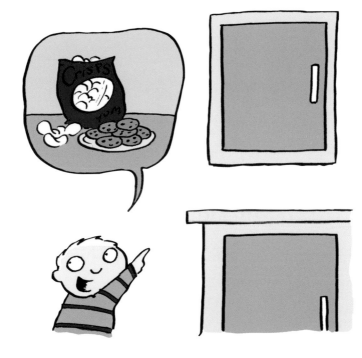

If your grandchild can crawl, remember to move breakable items out of its reach (and don't forget that a baby's reach can defy the laws of physics).

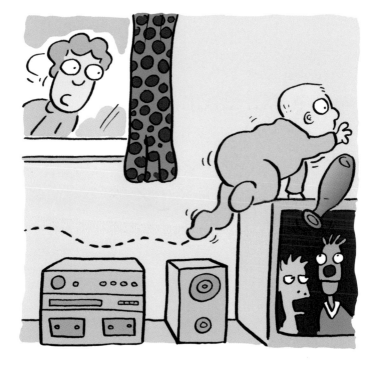

Having watched you putting DVDs in the machine's tray your grandchildren will be anxious to follow your example. Do not leave any round flat objects lying about – e.g. shortbread circles, Wagon Wheels, mini pizzas...

Early nights are very
important when your
grandchild comes to
stay. In order to survive,
you should probably be
in bed by about eight.

There is an unalterable law with babies. However fast asleep they may have been when they were left in their grandparents' care, within five minutes of their parents' departure they will be screaming.

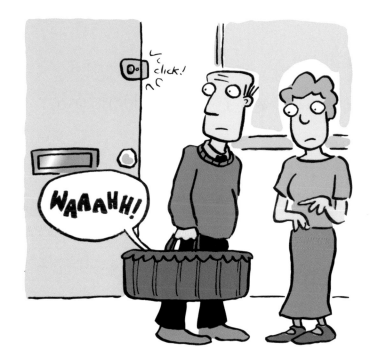

If your grandchildren come to stay with you during Potty Training, make sure you know the expressions which mean they *want to go.* This will save on your carpet-cleaning bill.

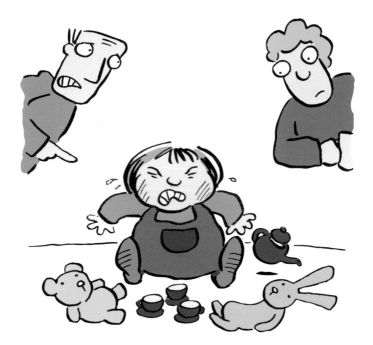

Though obviously you want all your friends and neighbours to see your grandchild, remember it is not a performing animal and may not do all its tricks to order.

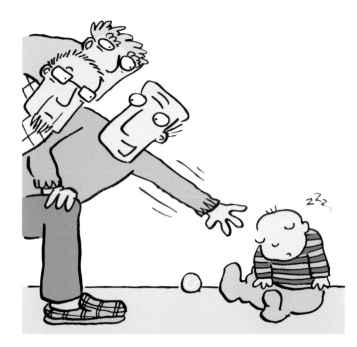

Some Disappointing Facts

Not every grandchild who does awfully good finger-painting will turn out to be the next Michelangelo.

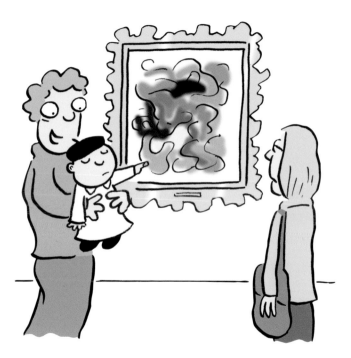

Nor does every baby who looks quite cute go on to become a supermodel.

Nor does every infant who is very good as an ox or ass in the school nativity play go on to become a Hollywood star.

Remarkable though it
may seem, the progress
of your grandchild's Potty
Training is not a topic
of universal interest.

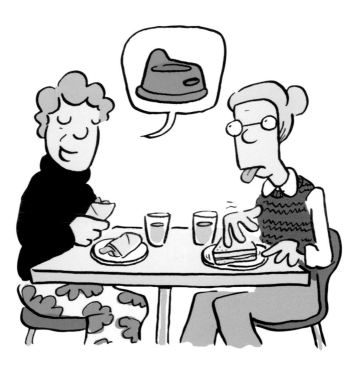

Family
Occasions

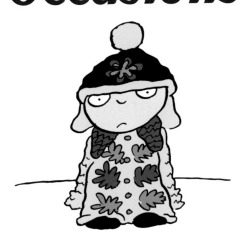

Picture Perfect

Every now and then
allow your grandchild
to do something without
taking a photograph of it.

Carry photographs to show at all times. People who claim not to be as interested in your grandchildren as you are must be joking.

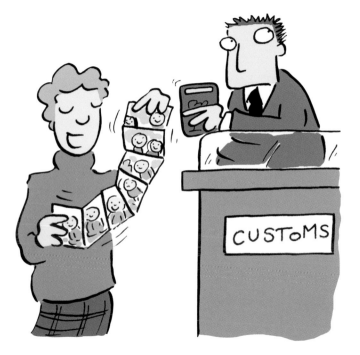

You can spend a very long time with your camera poised, waiting for a smile. And when you finally do press the shutter, you almost always miss it.

The invention of digital cameras means you don't have to get whole reels developed before you realise that your grandchild isn't smiling in any of the photos.

Babies don't understand
the concept of pointing.
If you want them to look
in a certain direction,
make a noise.

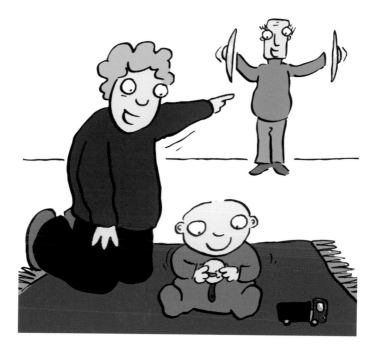

Don't embarrass your grandchildren by knitting for them. Unsuitable garments may not last, but photographs do.

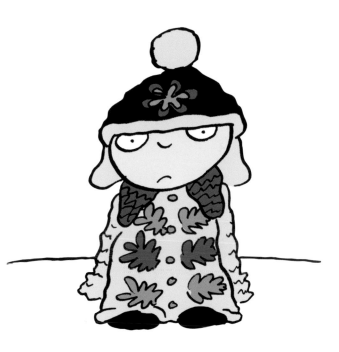

It is the obligation of every grandparent with a mobile phone to have a picture of a grandchild as wallpaper. This will mean that you coo every time you put your phone on.

Presents

If you do give a grandchild money, do not expect to get away with giving less the next time. They all have little calculators in their brains.

Be very careful when buying clothes for your grandchild's dolls. Giving the wrong garment can destroy your street cred forever.

Don't give your
grandchild a present
every time you see it.
Every now and then
play hard to get.

It is astonishing
the young age at
which grandchildren
will appreciate a
gift of money.

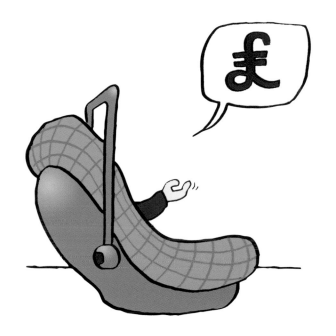

If you give your grandchild a present and get no thanks, avoid the instinct to ask, 'What do you say?' The child is quite likely to reply, 'Can I have another one?'

From a child's point
of view the word
'educational' on a toy
is the kiss of death.

Many parents disapprove
of their children
being given toy guns.
No children do.

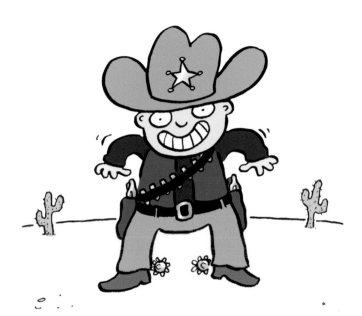

Giving your grandchildren
presents that make
irritating noises is not
fair on their parents...
but it is quite fun.

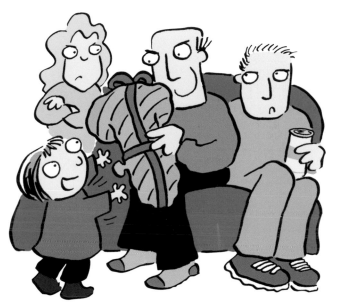

Don't worry if your grandchild ignores your present and plays with the one given by the other set of grandparents: it plays with yours when they visit.

Nursery Rhymes

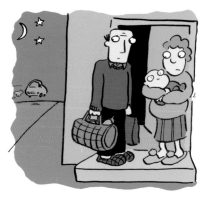

You probably grew up with nursery rhymes, but today's children are not so likely to hear them. It is therefore important that you keep the tradition alive. Some of the old rhymes, though, may need a little updating, as in these examples...

Jack Sprat could
eat no fat,
His wife could eat no lean;
And so he put her
on a diet –
Obesity's obscene.

Ding, dong, bell,
Pussy's in the well.
Who put her in?
One of those nasty
children who you must
never play with.

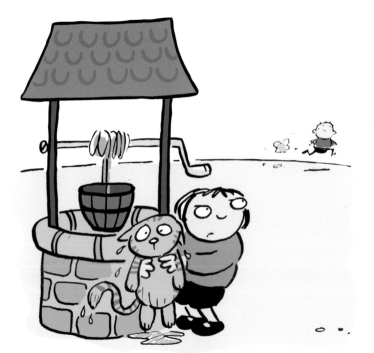

Old King Cole
Was a merry old soul,
And a merry old
soul was he,
He called for his pipe,
To the pub took a stroll,
But he couldn't smoke
in the Fiddlers Three.

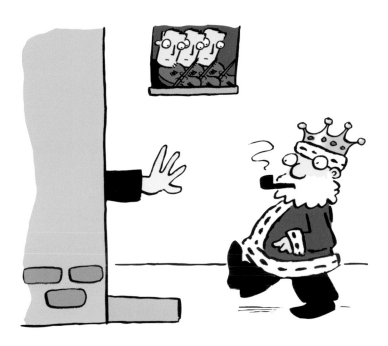

Jack and Jill went
up the hill
To fetch a pail of water.
Jack fell down and
broke his crown,
And sued Jill for
negligence after.

Mary, Mary, quite contrary,

How does your
garden grow?

With silver bells, and
cockle shells,

And lots of other stuff
recommended in a
television gardening show.

And a final thought...

Never say 'I'm not just a cheap baby-sitting service.' The fact is, you are.

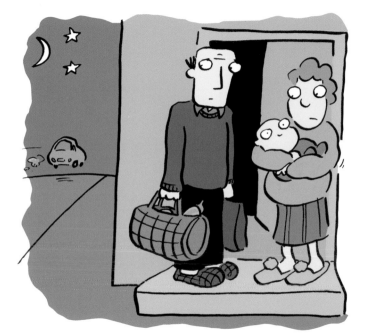

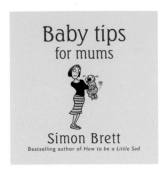

Baby tips
for mums

Simon Brett
Bestselling author of *How to be a Little Sod*

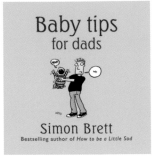

Baby tips
for dads

Simon Brett
Bestselling author of *How to be a Little Sod*

Whether you are a new mum or the seasoned father of a lively horde, make these little books the latest additions to your household.

www.summersdale.com